Acupressure

A Self-Care Guide for 10 Common Ailments

HUGH S. ALLEN

CONTENTS

	Introduction	1
1	Why Acupressure?	4
2	Acupressure for Quick Pain Relief	13
3	Acupressure for Arthritis	33
4	Acupressure for Stress & Muscle Tension	36
5	Acupressure for Anxiety & Trauma	41
6	Acupressure for Depression	44
7	Acupressure for Motion Sickness & Nausea	50
8	Acupressure for Weight Loss	56
9	Acupressure to Maintain & Restore Beauty	61
10	Acupressure for Sexual & Reproductive Health	65
11	Acupressure in Pregnancy	70
	Conclusion	77

INTRODUCTION

Are you always suffering from headaches, stomach aches, skin breakouts and other health issues? Are you tired of using every pill, tablet, gel and balm imaginable? If so, then it's time to try acupressure.

Acupressure or *Shiatsu* is a traditional method of healing that has been practiced by the Chinese for thousands of years. This healing art has gained popularity worldwide in the past two decades due to its efficacy in treating a variety of health problems. With all the accompanying side-effects of many traditional medicines, probably the most appealing reason for trying acupressure is that it does not make use of any drugs in the process of healing. There are no known side effects when practiced appropriately and consistent practice causes no harm.

Acupressure makes use of the fingers to apply pressure to various energy points in the body to activate and treat different organs and body parts. It can be used to target migraines, acne, kidney, liver, reproductive health issues, emotional and psychological concerns among others and it is appropriate for treatment of persons of all ages, from children to seniors. Use of this therapy is also very popular as it is painless, safe, inexpensive, easy to perform and requires little time.

Acupressure can give instant relief from migraines and back pains just by triggering the right energy points using the fingers. You can learn these techniques and relieve yourself from different ailments without waiting for long hours at the hospital and without incurring huge medical bills. Most of these techniques can even be performed on your own and you no longer have to wait for help from friends or family members. This also minimizes the use of traditional medicine to a great extent which is very beneficial.

An added advantage of using this form of healing is that it is a natural relaxant. The practice of acupressure relaxes the mind and the body which is vital for good health. The techniques are presented here in a succinct and straightforward way to enable you to follow easily and with great success. As you begin to practice, refer frequently to the chapters which relate to your particular need. This will be your ongoing guide to optimize the benefits to be gained from acupressure.

So why wait? Immerse yourself in these techniques and find relief from your aches and pain today!

1

WHY ACUPRESSURE?

Acupressure originated in China, but is currently practiced worldwide due to the popularity gained throughout centuries of practice. It has proven to be very effective in treating physical as well as psychological health issues. The therapy involves curing various ailments by triggering certain energy points in the body when slight pressure is applied with the fingers. The theory behind its effectiveness is that by stimulating the energy points, it releases negative thoughts and energy blocks from your being. It has proven to be very effective in treating physical as well as psychological health issues and can yield the following results when practiced:

- Release tension and stress
- Increase circulation
- Reduce or eliminate physical pain

- Effectively address sexual and reproductive issues
- Incorporate spirituality for holistic healing
- Improve overall health

The practice maintains that the body is classified into different meridians and trigger points.

- There are twelve main meridians, two sub-meridians and hundreds of points. The twelve main meridians are called the Yin-Yang or the primary meridians.

- The arm has Yin meridians that are associated with the heart, lung and pericardium (the membrane enclosing the heart). The Yang meridians of the arm are associated with the two intestines namely, the large intestine and the small intestine, along with the *triple burner* which is the term used in Chinese medicine to refer to the energy system which regulates the activities of other heat-generating organs.

- The Yin meridian of the leg deals with the spleen, kidney and liver; and the Yang meridians of the leg are associated with the stomach, urinary bladder and gall bladder.

- The sub-meridians or the extraordinary meridian differs from the main or the standard Yin Yang meridians as they are not directly associated with the organs, but only with the storage vessels or air passages.

- There are approximately 365 trigger points and they are spread across the entire body. The meridians are the pathways that connect the different points as well as the internal organs. These meridians are very similar to the blood vessels in function. As the blood vessels supply blood to the different organs, similarly the meridians carry the electrical energy or the spiritual energy throughout the body. They are known for their ability to connect the emotional, sensory and physiological elements of the body.

When these meridians and trigger points are worked on with gentle yet firm pressure using the fingers, muscular tension and any associated problem is alleviated. A thorough understanding of the trigger points and a good way to stimulate them can help to reduce pain and treat various health concerns even as a preventative measure. Acupressure is a great method of self-massage for anyone because it promotes good health even in the absence of pain or known malady.

Like acupressure, *acupuncture* uses the same basic principle of targeting the points across the body to treat pain, however, they are quite different in their use of tools. In acupressure, the fingers are the only 'tools' used to stimulate the points and meridians whereas needles and sharp objects are used for the same purpose in the practice of acupuncture. Acupuncture is a more invasive therapy and does require the expertise of a trained acupuncturist.

Comparatively, acupressure is a safer method of treating various medical issues because it does not require the use of any medications and tools or even potentially painful dangerous procedures like surgeries and operations.

Key Benefits of Acupressure

1. **Takes care of your overall well-being.** Acupressure is used to release the flow of the blocked passages in our body system so that the energy "Qi" or "Chi" can be effectively circulated throughout the body. This helps to maintain the overall well-being of the body keeping it fit and healthy.

2. **Accelerates the healing process.** Acupressure directly targets the meridians and energy channels associated with pain. Hence, the healing process can be much faster than using other treatments.

3. **Eliminates pain.** Pain in any part of the body can disrupt your regular activities, reduce your income-earning potential, and prevent you from functioning normally. This pain can be easily treated by acupressure.

4. **Makes you feel calm and relaxed.** Acupressure works on emotional and psychological issues like stress, anxiety, frustration, anger, moodiness and depression. The most common reason for these problems is a blocked energy channel or meridian. When the correct points are triggered, it facilitates the circulation of "Qi" or "Chi" energy in the body which relaxes the mind. This helps us to maintain

our composure even on intense, stress-filled days.

5. **Improves the skin and muscle tone.** The flow of energy in the body helps to rejuvenate and relax the skin and muscles, thereby improving the skin texture and muscle tone.

6. **Improves sex life.** Acupressure can solve many sex-related issues with some very simple techniques. When the points corresponding to these issues are stimulated properly, pelvic tension may be released and the most common problems are resolved.

7. **Enhances blood circulation.** When pressure points are properly stimulated, they activate the opening of blood channels which promote the flow of blood. When there is proper blood circulation, organs begin to functioning properly and other bodily functions are enhanced.

8. **Releases the build-up muscle tension.** The tension that is trapped in stiff muscles can be easily released by triggering the appropriate pressure points of the body. This helps in making the muscles fit and flexible.

9. **Minimizes the intake of drugs.** Our go-to solution for headaches and stomach aches is traditional drugs. These drugs, whether prescribed or over-the-counter, may provide instant relief, but may not be safe for long-term use. By adopting the practice of acupressure, you can minimize the use of these medicines considerably or perhaps even eliminate them.

10. **Safe, inexpensive cure**. Once you have a thorough understanding of acupressure, it can be performed on your own without even visiting a therapist. A working knowledge of the pressure points for different health problems can help you to get relief

quicker and in the privacy of your own home.

Caution: People who are suffering from any serious health conditions like heart disease, cancer and other life-threatening diseases should not perform this massage. Pregnant women should also be extra careful while triggering some points as it can induce labor early and also cause uterine contractions. People who have broken bones or fractures and slip discs should refrain from this technique as triggering the wrong points with insufficient knowledge can worsen the condition. If you have any open wound or fresh marks of surgery, then it is best to avoid the practice of acupressure altogether until the injuries and wounds are completely healed. The best thing to do in such cases is to contact your regular physician and discuss the possibilities and risks related to your condition. Only after getting approval from your doctor, should you start acupressure therapy.

2

ACUPRESSURE FOR QUICK PAIN RELIEF

Acupressure can either be performed independently or with the help of a trained acupressure therapist to treat all of the most common types of pain.

Back Pain

Back pain is one of the most common ailments that afflict people and can affect anyone, from young adults to seniors. Pain may be due to various reasons like slip discs, arthritis, sore muscles, sport injuries etc. and is typically treated with chiropractic massage, physical therapy or surgery. Using acupressure, there are many points in the hands and feet which can be triggered to get relief from back pain. Several studies have shown that the practice of acupressure has been more effective in providing quick, lasting relief for back pain than regular physical therapy.

There are three methods can be used to treat back pain:

1)   Triggering the points in the hand (joining of the valley)

- Sit in a comfortable position and ensure that your hands and feet are resting freely so that the pressure points can be stimulated properly.
- Gently place your right hand in the left hand.
- The first point lies in the region just below the thumb where the index finger and thumb meet on the web-like portion of skin.
- Place your left thumb firmly at this point.

- Place your left index finger at the bottom of the same point and press firmly while applying pressure.
- There will be a slight burning sensation or pain when you initially start applying the pressure at that point.
- This pinching pain indicates that you are stimulating the right spot.
- This pain will disappear after a couple of minutes and will be less painful as you stimulate the points more often.
- Count from one to ten or simply hold this pressure point firmly for ten seconds.
- Then slowly release the pressure and relax your fingers.
- Repeat the same routine two more times and hold it for about ten seconds each.
- Relax this hand and repeat the same procedure with the other hand as well.

2) Triggering the points in the foot (the point is also known as grandfather-grandson point, Gong sun or SP4)

- Sit in a comfortable position so that you can hold your foot in your hands.
- If you are unable to do this by yourself, ask someone to help you to stimulate the pressure point of the foot.
- If you have more pain on one side of the body, start by working on the foot corresponding to the more painful side.
- Locate the region on the foot in between the big toe and the second toe just below the area where these two bones meet.
- Keep your thumb at that particular position and your index finger just opposite or on the other side of the same spot.
- Firmly press this spot with both the fingers for one minute while taking deep breaths

- Slowly release the pressure, rub the spot and repeat the same method two to three times
- Then repeat the same procedure on the other foot as well

3) Triggering the points in the elbow (crooked pond/marsh)

- Place your arm in a slightly elevated position either with the help of an arm rest or simply by resting one arm over the other
- Begin the massage on the side of the body that has the most pain and stimulate the elbow on that side
- Next, locate the center of the crease that runs horizontally on the inside of your elbow
- Then place the thumb of the other hand, over the point in such a way that the other fingers of the hand wrap around the inner side of the elbow

- Apply a slight pressure over this particular spot in a motion towards the outside of the arm
- Hold this particular spot and continue the motion until you experience a twinge or pinching pain in that particular area
- Once the pain begins, it means that you have successfully identified the pressure spot
- Press firmly over this point for about one minute while taking deep breaths
- You can even increase the pressure if you are comfortable with the pain
- Slowly loosen the applied pressure, relax the point and slightly rub the area
- Continue this technique a couple more times on the same elbow
- Repeat this procedure on the other elbow as well
- Follow this acupressure routine at least once a week to achieve faster relief

Neck pain

Neck pain can be caused by many reasons including a poor sleeping position, a slouched back or even by some random activity like improperly balancing a cellular phone while talking. This is a fairly common issue, but can result in excruciating, ongoing pain if not treated. Using acupressure, neck pain can be treated easily in just a few minutes. The technique is simple and can be performed anywhere quickly and without much fuss. There are six important points across the body that can be stimulated to get relief from neck pain.

1. **Forehead.** This pressure point is called *"the drilling bamboo"*. It is a set of two points that are found on the forehead in the region where the ridge of the nose meets the bridge of the eyebrows. Press this area firmly for about a minute so you feel a slight pinching pain. Rub the spots in circular motions gently using your

fingers and continue doing this until you feel relief.

2. **Upper Neck.** This point is called "***the wind mansion***" and is found on the back of the neck just below the skull. You can feel a slight hollow or indentation in the center of that region when you move your fingers over the area. The pressure point lies within that indentation. When pressure is applied to that particular spot, it gets stimulated and works on the neck pain. So, press the spot with your index finger firmly for about one minute while taking deep breaths simultaneously. Gently release the pressure. Repeat this until you feel that the pain has subsided.

3. **Lower neck.** This point is called "***the gates of consciousness***". There are two pressure points located at the base of the skull on either side, in the hollow indentation between the two

vertical neck muscles. When these two spots are triggered, stiff and achy necks are relieved quickly.

4. **Sides of the neck.** This point is known as "***the window of heaven***". These are two points situated on either side of the neck, at the base of the skull in the indentations just about two inches away from the lobes of the ear. These two points can be stimulated by applying constant pressure at the points while rubbing the area in circular motion with the fingers. Continue applying pressure to the area until the pain subsides.

5. **Middle of the neck.** These two points are situated on the back of the neck, just below the skull about one inch away from the spine on either side. These two points are present in the thick rope-like muscles that run vertically down the neck. This point is known as "***the heavenly pillar***". These two points can be stimulated with the

thumb or index finger and pressed until relief is attained.

6. **Shoulder.** There are two points for neck pain, one on each shoulder called ***"the heavenly rejuvenation"***. These points are located in the well of the shoulder just about one or two inches away from the highest point of the shoulder. When the pressure is applied to these points, they get stimulated and minimize the pain or cure it completely. Pregnant women should not stimulate these points as it can induce a premature labor.

Headache

Headaches are probably the most common and frequently occurring pain that we experience. People generally reach for traditional medicines that are readily available. Though these drugs may cure recurring pain easily, many traditional drugs have known side-effects which can have a negative impact on us in the long run. One great way to avoid these potential side-effects and still cure the headaches is by using the method of acupressure. It releases the energy blockages and facilitates the circulation of energy in the body. It also releases certain endorphins that act as natural pain-killers to target and get rid of pain. The different points which can be stimulated to get relief from headaches are:

1. **Forehead.** There is a point in the region of the forehead called "***the third eye***" in between the two eyebrows. When this point is stimulated by applying constant pressure with the thumb or the index finger it will cause a pinching pain. Maintain the pressure for about one minute taking deep breaths then gently release the pressure. Do this continuously until the pain subsides.

2. **Hand.** The web-like fold of skin in between the thumb and the forefinger has a point called "***joining***

the valley" and is an excellent spot for treating headaches. Press this spot firmly using the thumb and index finger of the opposite hand for about one minute until you experience a pinching pain. Take some deep breaths while you apply pressure to the spot. Gently release the pressure and continue until the pain subsides. Repeat the same with the opposite hand for extra relief.

3. **Neck.** There are two points at the back of the neck called "*the gates of consciousness*" which can be stimulated for getting relief from headaches. Place your fingers on the back of your neck just below the skull. Move your finger from the center of the neck to about two to three inches towards the side until you come across an indentation on either side of the neck. Slightly tilt your head towards the back and stimulate these points using the thumb or the index

finger. Press firmly in the indented area for about two minutes until you begin to feel better.

4. **Head.** The pressure point lies on top of the head and it can be located by creating an imaginary line that runs from ear to ear over the head. Create another imaginary line that starts from the middle of your forehead that runs over the head until it reaches the midpoint of the first imaginary line. The point of intersection is the pressure point that needs stimulation. Press this point firmly using the forefinger/index finger continuously for about one minute, taking deep breaths. Continue pressing the point until the pain stops.

5. **Foot.** This pressure point is called *"the bigger rushing"* and is situated in the region between the big toe and the second toe of the foot towards the top. Pinch this point firmly while

applying pressure and also rub the area with your thumb in a circular motion for one minute. Take a deep breath while pressing the spot and release it. Continue doing this until you get some relief from your pain and repeat the same procedure for the other foot as well.

Other Physical Pain

Acupressure has also been found to be a safe and inexpensive solution to other types of physical pain. It can be used to treat toothaches, ear aches, eye strains and stomach aches among others.

Toothaches. This pain can be reduced or cured by stimulating the points given below. There are four major points that deal with toothaches:

- The first point is called "***the facial beauty***" and is located on the face, just below the cheek bone. This point lies in the line directly below the pupil of the eye.

- The second point "**the jaw chariot**" lies just in front of the ear lobe in between the upper and lower jaw. The muscles at this point bulge when the back teeth are clenched.
- The third point is "**the shoulder meeting point**" and is situated at the base of the upper arm about one inch towards the back and two inches up towards the shoulder. This point is situated on the outer part of the arm.
- The fourth point is called "**the joining of the valley**" and is located in the webbing between the index finger and the thumb. The muscle that bulges when both fingers are brought close together contains the pressure point.

All these points contribute in relieving the toothaches, dental neuralgia and other dental issues.

Ear-aches. There are five points that can be stimulated to reduce pain in the ear:

- There is a point called "**the ear gate**" just outside of the opening of the ear in an indentation. This hollow will deepen when the mouth is open.
- The second point is "**the listening place**" situated just about an inch above the first point.
- The third point called "**the reunion of hearing**" lies about one inch below the first point.
- The fourth point is "**the windscreen**" which lies within the hollow indentation behind the ear lobe.
- The fifth point is "**the bigger stream**" that is present in the ankle region in between the Achilles tendon and the ankle bone towards the back.

Stimulating these points helps in relieving ear pains, hearing problems, ear blocks, itchy ears and pressure in the ear.

Eye strain. There are seven main points that can be stimulated to get relief from strained or pained eyes:

- The first point is "*the third eye*" that lies in the center of the forehead in between the two eyebrows. This point is exactly located in the region of the third eye or the point where the bridge of the nose meets the forehead.
- The second point is called "*the drilling bamboo*" and lies at the inner tip of the eyebrows in the small indentations just outside the nose bridge. This particular point can be stimulated to get relief from various eye problems like foggy or blurry vision, pain and redness of the eyes and itching in the eyes.
- The third point is "*the four whites*" which is situated in the indentation of the cheek bones, about one inch below the center of the lower eye ridge.

- The fourth point is "*the facial beauty*" located just below the cheek bone in the same line as the pupil of the eye.
- The fifth point is called "*the wind mansion*" and is situated at the base of the skull in the hollow indentation at the top of the spine.
- The sixth point is called "*the heavenly pillar*" and is located at the back of the neck, at the base of the skull on the rope-like muscles that are found about an inch on either side of the spine.
- The last point is on the foot, at the region of the webbing between the big toe and the second toe. The center of this webbing has the pressure point called "*the bigger rushing*".

All of these points can be stimulated by applying constant pressure for about a minute while taking deep breaths. When this method is used regularly most common eye complaints can be alleviated or completely eliminated.

Stomach pain. There are six points that can be stimulated using the acupressure technique to get relief from stomach pains. These six points concentrate mainly on treating the stomach:

- One point is called the "***center of power***" and is situated in the center of the body on the midline, in between the base of the breast bone and the belly button.
- The next point is called "***the sea of energy***" and is situated about two to three centimeters below the navel region.
- The third point is called "***the three-mile point***" and is located about three finger-widths below the knee cap, towards the outside, just off the shin bone.
- The fourth and the fifth sets of points are situated in the lower back region, between the second and the third lumbar vertebrae about an inch away from the spine. These points are called "***the sea of vitality***".

- The sixth point is situated about one thumb width below the ball of the foot, towards the heel region and is called **"the grandfather-grandson"** or the **"Gong sun point"**.
- The seventh point is **"the inner gate"** and is situated on the wrist of the hand about two fingers width below the crease, in the center.

All these points help in treating the various problems associated with the stomach like improper digestion, acidity, nausea, indigestion, constipation, diarrhea and stomach aches.

3

ACUPRESSURE FOR ARTHRITIS

This is one of the most painful medical conditions, it involves inflammation and pain in the muscle and bones of the joints. The pain can be caused due to a number of factors such as injuries, excessive physical activity, obesity or genetics. There is a wide range of treatments available for treating arthritis like massage, physical therapy and surgery. Acupressure is also an effective way of achieving relief. The pressure points that are to be stimulated to activate the appropriate energy channels are:

1. **Elbow.** This point is called *"the crooked pond"* and is situated in the elbow crease towards the upper edge. This point helps in curing arthritic pain that occurs in the shoulder and elbow.

2. **Arm.** This point is situated about four centimeters above the wrist in the center region between the two bones i.e. radius and ulna and is known as **"*the outer gate*"**. Stimulating this point helps to provide relief from rheumatoid arthritis.

3. **Hand**. This point is called "***the joining of the valley***" and is situated in the webbing between the thumb and the index finger. Pinch the middle of this webbing firmly with the help of the thumb and forefinger of the opposite hand to get relief from the pain. Pregnant women should avoid this point as it can induce labor. This point will help in getting relief from arthritic pains in the knee and shoulders.

4. **Knee.** This point is called "***the three-mile point***" and is situated about four finger-widths below the kneecap just off the shin bone towards the outside. Stimulating this point regularly is very

important as it can help to overcome the fatigue caused by the arthritic pain and strengthens the joints and muscles.

5. **Upper neck.** There is a set of two points called "**the gates of consciousness**" that are present at the base of the skull in the indentation between the two thick long muscles. They are present on either side of the spine about two-three inches apart from each other depending upon the size of the head. Stimulating these points helps to overcome the pains commonly associated with arthritis, such as headaches, insomnia, irritability, fatigue, muscle and joint pains.

4

ACUPRESSURE FOR STRESS & MUSCLE TENSION

This is an almost unavoidable by-product of our modern lifestyle. Men and women alike are required to manage the demands of their work and personal lives but most of have not yet achieved that work/life balance that is necessary. It has become increasingly difficult and frustrating to bring our best selves to our family and personal responsibilities after spending 8-10 hours in the office glued to the desk or computer. This hectic lifestyle fosters anxiety and stress that expresses itself through muscle pain and stiffness. These problems may be treated using reflexology and acupressure. There are several points in the body which can be stimulated for stress relief and to improve energy circulation in the body.

1. **Leg**. This part consists of a point called "***the three-mile point***" and is

situated about three finger-widths below the kneecap, towards the outside and just off the shin bone. Apply constant pressure at this point for about a minute and take deep breaths along with it. Slowly release the point and repeat for extra relief.

2. **Foot**. There are two points in the foot region. The first point is called "the greater rushing" and is located in the webbing between the big toe and the second toe. Applying pressure at this point helps to unblock the energy passages and facilitates proper energy circulation throughout the meridians. The second point is "***the grandfather–grandson***" point or "***the Gong sun***" point that is located towards the inner surface of the foot about three finger-widths below the base of the big toe. Stimulating this point regularly for about one minute helps to free the mind of anxiety.

3. **Forearm.** There are two points here that help in overcoming stress. The first point is the "***inner gate***" which is situated almost in the center about three to four finger-widths below the wrist crease towards the elbow. Stimulate this point by pressing the spot firmly while taking deep breaths to eliminate stress and worry.

   a. The other point is "***the outer gate***" that is located on the back side of the arm, in between the two tendons, about four finger-widths above the wrist towards the elbow. This point helps in enhancing the energy flow in the body and also nourishes the immune system.

4. **Hand.** The hand consists of a point in the webbing between the thumb and the index finger. This point is called the "***joining of the valley***" and is used

to minimize muscle tension and eliminate stress.

5. **Chest.** This point is called "***the central treasury***" and is situated on the sides of the body in the region about two fingers width above the spot where the arms meet the chest. Stimulating this point regularly helps to balance the emotions and manage stress levels.

6. **Lower back.** There is a set of two points called "***the wills chamber***" that is situated in the waist region about three finger-widths away from the spine on either side. Triggering this point helps to ease out the muscle tension in the back and aid in proper energy circulation through the meridians.

7. **Shoulders.** There is a point called "***the heavenly rejuvenation***" that is located on each of the shoulders

midway between the base of the neck and the ridge of the shoulder. Stimulating this point helps in releasing stress and tension from the muscles and aids in the unhindered flow of energy.

5

ACUPRESSURE FOR ANXIETY & TRAUMA

People very often suffer from trauma and anxiety which may be caused due to a number of reasons. Some common ways to treat this psychological issue is through drugs, therapy, counseling and meditation. Using acupressure in this scenario involves the stimulation of a few pressure points so that the blocked energy channels are released and the anxiety and trauma are eliminated from the system.

1. **Neck.** There is a set of two points situated at the base of the skull on the ropy muscles that are found about an inch away from the spine. This point is called "***the heavenly pillar***" and helps in getting over trauma, anxiety, feelings of depression and insomnia.

2. **Shoulders**. There is a set of two points situated on each shoulder called "***the shoulder well***". The points are located in between the base of the neck and the outer end of the shoulders about two inches below the top of the shoulder. This is a great spot to stimulate to achieve relief from anxiety and trauma.

3. **Elbow**. The point in this part is called the "***the crooked marsh***" situated towards the inner side of the arm near the lower side of the elbow crease, when the arm is bent. This point is good for relieving anxiety and its associated problems.

4. **Arm.** This point is situated at the center about two inches away from the wrist crease towards the inner side of the forearm and is known as "***the inner gate***". This point helps to provide relief from palpitations, trauma and anxiety. There is another

point situated on the forearm towards the side of the pinky finger called "**the spirit gate**". This point lies in the indentation that occurs near the crease of the wrist. It helps to overcome fear, anxiety, stress, trauma and emotional imbalance.

5. **Forehead**. This point is situated in between the two eyebrows in the middle of the forehead at the region of the third eye and is called as "**the third eye point**". This point helps in calming the body from trauma, nervousness and anxiety.

6. **Chest**. This point is situated at the center of the breast bone about three to four centimeters above the base of the breast bone. This point is called the "**sea of tranquility**". Stimulating this point helps to overcome nervousness, anxiety, depression, hysteria and trauma.

6

ACUPRESSURE FOR DEPRESSION

Depression and other emotional problems can also be treated using acupressure. While there are other treatments that assist with overcoming depression, acupressure is a quick and safe way as it deals directly with the release of the blocked air channels. When the air channels are unblocked, energy travels throughout the system slowly driving out the vestiges of depression and incorporating freshness and cheerfulness in the body.

1. **Head and neck.** The back of the upper neck region consists of two sets of points that can help in overcoming depression. The first set of points is called **_the gates of consciousness_** and is located just at the base of the skull in the hollow indentation

between the two thick vertical neck muscles. These two points are about two to three inches apart from each other depending on the size of the head.

The second set of points is called the "**heavenly pillar**". It is also located at the base of the skull, about one inch below the first set of points and about one inch on either side of the spine, on the ropy muscles. Both these sets of points help in relieving distress, emotional pain and depression when stimulated.

2. **Back.** This point is called "**the vital diaphragm**" and is located on either side of the spine at the level of the heart, in between the shoulder blades. Stimulating this point regularly helps to get relief from emotional imbalance, grief and depression.

3. **Lower back.** There are two sets of points called *"the sea of vitality"* which are located in the lower back region in between the second and the third lumbar vertebrae, about an inch away from the spine. Be careful not to press on these points firmly if suffering from slip discs, injured back, or fractured bones.

4. **Forehead.** The point is located in the region of the third eye in the center region in between the two eyebrows. This spot can be stimulated by pressing firmly with the index finger or thumb for about one minute each time. This helps to overcome problems such as depression, emotional imbalance and anxiety.

5. **Chest.** This region consists of three main points:

- There is one point called "***elegant mansion***" that is situated just below the collar bone, in the indentation above the first rib and outside the upper breast bone. This point also relieves from anxiety and depression.
- There is another set of points called "***letting go***" located in the upper chest region, about five centimeters above the crease of the armpit. These points relieve depression, repressed emotions, grief and sorrow.
- The last sets of points in the chest region lie at the center of the breast bone just about four cm away from the base of the breast bone. These points are called "***sea of tranquility***" and they help in alleviating depression, grief, hysteria and other symptoms of emotional imbalance.

6. **Knee.** The point for counteracting depression is called "***the three-mile point***" and it lies about four finger-

widths below the knee cap, just off the shin bone. This point helps in fighting depression and other negative emotions.

7. **Top of the head.** There are three points in this region that can be stimulated to get relief from depression:

- The first point is called the "**one hundredth point**" and it lies on top of the head right in the middle. You can even locate this point by moving your left finger from the left ear towards the top and the right finger from the right ear towards the top at a similar pace. The place where both the fingers meet is the pressure point.
- The second point called "**the anterior summit**" lies just about an inch in front of the first point.
- The third set of points called "**the posterior summit**" is situated about

one inch behind the first set of points. All of these three sets of points help in relieving depression and symptoms of emotional imbalance.

7

ACUPRESSURE FOR MOTION SICKNESS & NAUSEA

Nausea is a common part of life. It can occur while travelling, as a result of a hangover, during pregnancy, or simply from the smell of a potent odor like a sanitizer or even a cologne. Nausea is also well-known to be one of the more unpleasant side-effects of chemotherapy. While there are several other methods of treating nausea, acupressure is one of the safest and most inexpensive methods of treatment. Just by triggering a few points in our body, nausea can easily be controlled.

There are two ways of doing this massage, either by using the fingers or a wristband.

Fingers

- For this technique, relax your arms and position them in such a way that

the arms lie directly in front of you
with the palms facing upwards

- Be seated in a comfortable position, so that you can do this easily without much effort
- If you are working on the pressure points of the left hand, then place the three fingers of your other hand, at the region that lies just below the crease of the wrist
- Then place the thumb of the right hand just below the fingers in the place between the two tendons
- This is the pressure point that you need to stimulate and it is called "*the inner gate*" or *P6*
- The same point on the other side of the hand (opposite side) is called "*the outer gate*" or *SJ5*
- Then apply pressure to these points using your fingers
- Whenever you feel nauseated, just place your thumb and the index finger on either of these pressure points,

press firmly and gently rub in a circular motion
- This may be slightly painful initially
- This method will usually give immediate relief from nausea, but the results can also be delayed by about five or ten minutes
- You may also place both your wrists close to each other and tap them several times while taking deep breaths
- This tapping of the wrists may be easier for some people to attain relief than trying to find the accurate position of the pressure points

There is another trigger point just below the kneecap, which can be stimulated to achieve relief from nausea.

- To do this, place four fingers on the region just below the area of the knee cap
- Place the opposite hand just below the little finger that is already in position.

- You can test the accuracy of the point by moving your foot up and down. If the muscle at the point will flex, then it means that you have located the right point.
- This pressure point is called "*the three miles*" or the **ST36** point and is one of the most commonly used pressure points for boosting energy
- Apply pressure to that point firmly using your fingers and gently rub it up and down in the same region, hold it for a minute or so and release the tension
- Repeat the same method for the other knee as well for better relief

Wrist Bands

This technique makes use of an anti-nausea wristband that is available in pharmacies or online stores. These bands are designed to apply the optimum pressure to the correct points of the wrist. These bands usually carry a small knob or a button like a notch on the inner surface of the band that comes in contact with the pressure points. There are different types of bands available on the market featuring distinct fabric, color and styles.

If you do not wish to spend money on these ready-made bands then you can even prepare your own wristband. For this you will require a regular wrist band or a wrist watch and a small button or any small pebble or object. Just place this stone or object in the region of the pressure point and wear the wristwatch or band over it so that it stays firmly in place without moving.

After you wear the wrist band, find the exact location of the pressure point (refer to the above method for locating the point). Make sure that the stone or object that you place in the wrist band coincides with the point and is held firmly in place. Secure the wrist band so that it is not loose and does not move up and down the wrist or slide out of place. Ensure that you are feeling just enough pressure to the points - not too much or too little, but just enough to provide continual stimulation.

If the pain becomes too intense, loosen the band a bit. Once you are fully accustomed to the use of this band, you will have to press on the stone or knob of the band over the points with a little bit more pressure to get extra relief.

8

ACUPRESSURE FOR WEIGHT LOSS

Disproportionate body weight is an issue that affects a large percentage of the world population. People often make the assumption that an obese person is a glutton, however, there can be many reasons for weight gain, for example, elevated blood sugar levels, hormonal problems or an ineffective digestive system. In acupressure therapy, the key to losing weight is to stimulate the trigger points of the digestive system so that any failing of the digestion process can be rectified. This acupressure method when combined with a balanced diet and proper exercise can help to painlessly shed those extra pounds.

Before beginning this technique on your own, consult your general physician for advice on whether acupressure is right for you and if there are any possible associated risks. Only after a doctor's consultation should you opt for weight loss through acupressure.

There are different pressures points for weight loss located throughout the entire body:

1. **Ear.** There is an appetite control point situated on the fleshy flap (Tragus) of the ear, which is present above the ear lobe and in front of the ear canal. This pressure point has found to reduce or stop overeating when stimulated. So, when you apply a constant pressure at this point for about three minutes, the appetite point is stimulated which in turn prevents you from overeating. Do this on the other Tragus as well. Once the urge for overeating is minimized, the body consumes only the required amount of food. This helps you to manage your food intake.

2. **Ankle.** The pressure point for the spleen lies in the region just above the ankle bone. This spot is located on the

inner region of the ankle just off the bone. In other words, this point lies about four inches away from the center of the ankle bone. This pressure point helps to tighten the digestive system. Trigger this point with the help of your knuckles or thumb and apply pressure firmly on it for about one minute and gently release the pressure. If you are pregnant then you should not perform this method at all as there are chances of it inducing labor pains as well.

3. **Knee Cap.** The point that lies just below the knee cap on the shin bone is a pressure point for treating circulatory and digestive system issues. To locate this point, leave about four fingers gap from the lower point of the knee cap and about one inch off the shin bone away towards the outside. If the muscles in that spot flex when you move your leg up and down it means that you have located

the right point. Press this point firmly for about one minute and then slowly release it.

4. **Side of the leg.** This point is the one that targets the spleen and helps in the regulation of water metabolism in our body. This spot is fairly easy to locate. It lies on the inner surface of the leg in the rounded or hollowed fleshy part of the leg about one inch towards from the knee along the shin bone. In other words, it lies in the inner side of the leg, in-between the calf muscles and the shin bone about an inch below the knee. Apply pressure to this point firmly for about three minutes until you feel a pinching pain and gently release it.

5. **Elbow.** Lying near the elbow is the point called "***the crooked marsh***". This point is for targeting the large intestines. Sit in a comfortable position and begin the procedure with

the left hand first. Place the left hand close to the chest. With your right hand, leave about two fingers gap away from the elbow crease in the direction towards the wrist. Using the thumb of the right hand, firmly apply pressure to this spot for about one minute. Repeat this on the other arm as well for extra relief. Stimulating this pressure point will also help in eliminating the excess heat and moisture from the body and also maintain intestinal health.

9

ACUPRESSURE TO MAINTAIN & RESTORE BEAUTY

Acupressure can also be used to treat various skin conditions. There are several pressure points across the body which can treat these problems and improve the appearance. When these trigger points are stimulated, it enables proper energy flow to the body parts, facilitates the release of blocked passages and also minimizes the stress and tension in the muscles. This rejuvenates the skin and gives it a much younger, healthier appearance. It also minimizes or eliminates the incidence of pimples and acne.

1. **Neck.** There are two points called "***the heavenly pillar***" that are located at the back of the neck just below the skull, about an inch away on either side of the spine. They are present on

the rope-like vertical neck muscles to be exact. When these points are regularly stimulated by pressing them firmly for about a minute, they work on the muscles of the face and gives us relief from stress related skin problems like acne.

2. **Lower back.** There are two sets of points called "***the sea of vitality***" on the lower back in the region in between the second and the third lumbar vertebrae, about an inch away from either side of the spine. These points need not be pressed firmly, gently massaging or rubbing these points is sufficient to stimulate them. These points can improve the texture of the skin and also addresses problems such as eczema, acne, rashes, allergies and even surface bruises on the body.

3. **Forehead.** There is another point that helps in nourishing the skin. It is

located exactly centered between the two eyebrows and is called the "***third eye point***".

4. **Face.** This point is called "***four whites***" and is located on the face just about a finger-width below the lower ridge of the eye socket. It is present in the same line as the iris of the eye within the cheek indentation. Stimulating this point helps to overcome acne and blemishes on the face.

There is another point on the face called "***the facial beauty***" which is located just below the cheek bones. This point lies directly in line with the pupil of the eye. By stimulating this point regularly with optimum pressure, skin conditions like facial blemishes, scars, bruises, saggy cheeks, wrinkles and acne can be treated along with proper energy circulation in the face.

5. **Knee.** This point is called "*the three-mile point*" and it lies about four finger-widths below the knee cap, just off the shin bone. It helps in enhancing the skin conditions throughout the body along with improving the tone of muscles and skin.

6. **Ears.** There is a point called "*heavenly appearance*" on either side of the face just below the jaw bone and directly behind the ear lobe, which can be stimulated to improve the luster of the skin and also to get relief from hives.

    There is another point called "*windscreen*" in the small hollow indentation behind the ear, which also helps in improving the skin.

10

ACUPRESSURE FOR SEXUAL & REPRODUCTIVE HEALTH

Acupressure can also be used to treat some problems related to impotency, menstrual cramps, vaginal infections and infertility. These sexual and reproductive health problems can be caused due to a number of factors. For a person to be sexually healthy there must be a proper flow of energy in the pelvic area and the muscles should be tension-free and flexible and this can easily be achieved by using acupressure. There are several points that can be stimulated to treat problems in both male and female reproductive systems. All the points need not be stimulated at the same time. Stimulating one or two points regularly may be enough to treat any existing issue.

The pressure points for the pelvic region are:

1. **Sacral point.** The acupressure point lies in the sacral region just above the tail bone. Stimulate this point continuously for about a minute with the fingers. Do this regularly so that the blocked air passages are unblocked and energy is circulated throughout the pelvic area.

2. **Lower back points.** There are two sets of points called "*the sea of vitality*" in the lower back region between the second and third lumbar vertebrae to be precise. To locate these points, leave about two to four fingers-width gaps on either side of the spine. These points should lie on the same line as the belly button in the waist region. Stimulating these points regularly with the fingers can help in treating impotency, premature ejaculation and weak erections.

3. **Sole of the foot.** There is a point that lies on the sole of the foot almost in the

middle, between the two fleshy pads at the base of the ball of the foot called "***the bubbling springs***". Stimulating this point thoroughly using the thumb by pressing hard and rubbing the spot in circular motions will help to resolve the issues of impotency in men and hot flashes in menopausal women.

4. **Belly region.** This point is called "***the sea of energy***" and is very easy to locate. It is situated just three finger-widths below the belly button. Stimulating this point regularly with the fingers, help to minimize problems such as irregular periods and irregular vaginal discharge in women.

There is another point called "***the gate of origin***" that lies about four finger-widths directly below the belly button. Triggering this point also helps to relieve from urinary incontinence, irregular periods, and irregular vaginal discharge and also helps in strengthening the reproductive system.

5. **Pelvic region.** There are two sets of points in the pelvic region called "***the mansion cottage***" and "***the rushing door***". They are situated one below the other on either side, in the area of the crease where the leg and the trunk meet. These points can be stimulated regularly to get relief from problems such as menstrual cramps, abdominal discomfort and impotency.

6. **Leg.** There is a point called "***the three-mile point***" that is situated about four fingers widths below the knee cap just off the shin bone. If the muscle at that spot will flex when you move the leg up and down, it means that you have located the right spot. This spot needs to be stimulated regularly for several months to get relief from various sexual problems.

7. **Foot**. There is a point that lies in between the Achilles tendon and the ankle bone toward the inner surface of the leg called *"the bigger stream"*. Stimulating this point helps to rectify problems such as leakage of semen, irregular periods and sexual tension.

11

ACUPRESSURE IN PREGNANCY

Using the technique of acupressure, the process of labor can also be induced or accelerated. Most women prefer a natural induction of labor and this is one such technique that can be followed. By stimulating the pressure point for inducing labor, the cervix is encouraged to dilate as well as to produce contractions.

Pregnant women should never consider stimulating those pressure points that are associated with inducing labor until at least thirty-nine weeks of pregnancy is complete. This should be strictly followed as inducing labor too early poses a risk for mother and child. Even after passing the thirty-nine-week mark, any attempt to induce labor should be sanctioned by your physician beforehand.

The pressure points for inducing labor are located in the hand, neck, back, foot and ankle:

1. **Hand.** This point is also known as the ***Hokum*** or the ***"joining of the valley"*** and is one of the most commonly stimulated points to induce labor. This spot is present in the webbing between the index finger and the thumb. To apply this technique, follow the steps given below.

   - Start by pressing the webbing or the fold of skin firmly until you start to feel a pinching pain.
   - The point lies almost in the middle of the hand in between the first and the second Metacarpal bones.
   - Constantly apply pressure over that point and gently rub the same spot in a circular motion using your fingers.
   - When you feel too much pressure or the hand is tired, just shake the hands loose several times so that it relaxes and repeat the same method.

- Stop rubbing the point when you first start to feel the contraction.
- Once the contraction passes, resume the same step and pinch the webbing again.
- Stimulating this point over and over again helps in contracting the uterus and aids in descending the baby into the pelvic cavity.
- The stimulation of this point has also helped in easing out the pains during continuous contractions.

2. **Neck.** The point for gall bladder stimulation lies in the region between the neck and shoulder. This pressure point is also called the *Jian Jing* or the *gall bladder 21*. For performing this technique, follow these steps:
- Find the knob at the top of the spine and the ball in the region of the shoulder.
- The gall bladder 21 pressure point lies in the center, between these two points on each side.

- Slowly, yet firmly, apply pressure to this spot with the help of the thumb or the index finger in a downward motion.
- Hold this pressure point for about three minutes and gently release it.
- This point also induces labor and facilitates contractions.

3. **Back.** The lower back consists of a pressure point that is responsible for the proper functioning of the urinary bladder and is called the *ciliao* or the *bladder 32*. This pressure point is also used to induce labor in pregnant women, ease the pain of contractions and also help the baby to descend properly into the pelvic cavity.
- For this technique, the person who is pregnant is required to kneel down on the floor or a bed.
- The point is located on the lower back in between the lumbar spine and the dimple like hollow that is found in the lower back region.

- After you locate the spot in between the dimples, use your thumb or index finger to press firmly over the bladder 32 point.
- Apply pressure to the spot and rub it in a circular motion for about three minutes.
- If the hollow dimple is not located easily, just measure about one finger length from the buttock crease upwards and keep about one thumb width on either side of the spine.
- Stimulate this pressure point until you start developing contractions.

4. **Foot.** The point that is located on the foot, just above the ankle bone is called the **SP6, spleen 6** or the **Sanyinjiao** point. Stimulating this point will help in stretching the cervix and strengthening weak contractions.
- To locate this point, leave about three fingers distance above the shin bone.
- This point is found at the back of the leg just off the shin bone.

- This point will be very tender and is very sensitive in pregnant women.
- After you locate the point, apply firm pressure to this point by rubbing the spot in circles until a contraction is developed.
- Wait until each contraction passes and resume the same technique again.
- The pinky toe also is another point which can be stimulated for inducing labor and also to reposition breech babies.
- This point is known as the **Zhiyin** point or the **bladder 67**.
- To stimulate this point, place the pregnant woman's foot in your hand and firmly apply pressure to the tip of the pinky toe, just under the toenail. This will stimulate it and induce labor.

5. **Ankle.** This point is also called the **Kunlun** point or the **bladder 60** pressure point. This spot is usually stimulated in the initial stage of the

labor when the baby has not yet descended into the pelvic cavity.

- Start the procedure by locating this pressure point.
- It is found in the region between the ankle bone and the Achilles tendon.
- Apply pressure to the spot and rub it in a circular motion for about two minutes firmly and then release it.
- This helps in relieving the pain during contractions and induces labor.

12

CONCLUSION

In modern society, we have many alternative therapy methods available to us to address our health concerns. In the last two decades we have seen the emergence of many holistic health clinics as well as yoga and meditation centers. Their growth and popularity are evidence that people are seeking holistic alternatives to traditional health care.

The core theme common to these 'new' therapies is relaxing the body and calming the mind with the primary focus being to maintain the overall well-being of the individual. With the increased stress and the associated health problems of our modern lifestyle, these therapies play a key role in overcoming ailments whose incidence have risen to unprecedented levels. Stress and anxiety have created monsters that traditional medicine cannot defeat without using drugs whose strength combats the problem but creates problems of its own. This is the reason alternative therapies have grown and will continue to grow in popularity.

Acupressure has risen to prominence as one of the safest and least invasive ways to achieve relief from various health problems. In practice, it involves knowing the pressure points and the associated organs and the only tools required are the fingertips to stimulate these points. The mechanism behind its success is the release of energy blocks in the different meridians. When these energy passages are unblocked, proper circulation of "*Qi*" energy can take place which facilitates the proper functioning of the organs as well as better blood circulation.

Perhaps acupressure's greatest advantage is in its simplicity – anyone can find their pressure points and regularly stimulate them to improve their health. As you have read, many of the energy points can positively impact multiple areas of the body so in targeting one area, you can be improving your health in others as well. With no known side-effects of this technique, it can be used by anyone to achieve better health in multiple areas. Whether you use acupressure to enhance your overall wellness by addressing skin condition, appearance or weight loss; or you use it to treat physical or psychological problems like stress, depression, infertility or chronic pain; acupressure can also be integrated into your regular self-care routine. With the right ambience, it can be a soothing therapy to relax your mind and body while it administers healing to the whole *you*.

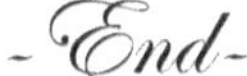

- End -

ABOUT THE AUTHOR

Hugh Allen is a self-proclaimed social scientist who has long been fascinated with the mind and its power to effect change. This led him to study eastern healing practices for many years and he is a firm believer in their ability to restore health and wellness.

He has practiced meditation for over fifteen years and leads an informal group of meditation and yoga enthusiasts. In his spare time, Hugh collects vintage music and music paraphernalia and is a regular at local flea markets and estate sales.

BOOKS BY HUGH S. ALLEN

- Meditation: The Beginner's Guide to Serenity

- Mindfulness for Beginners

- Pain Management